The Diagnosis Is Terminal

What Do We Do Now?

**A guide to help manage the journey
through terminal illness**

80% of you need 80% of this information
20% of you need 20% of this information

None of us know it all
If you can use one item it will be worth your effort

JIM M. COSTON, JR.

WESTBOW
PRESS®
A DIVISION OF THOMAS NELSON
& ZONDERVAN

WestBow Press books may be ordered through booksellers or by contacting:

WestBow Press
A Division of Thomas Nelson & Zondervan
1663 Liberty Drive
Bloomington, IN 47403
www.westbowpress.com
1 (866) 928-1240

ISBN: 978-1-5127-1279-7 (sc)
ISBN: 978-1-5127-1280-3 (e)

Library of Congress Control Number: 2015915162

Print information available on the last page.

WestBow Press rev. date: 09/30/2015

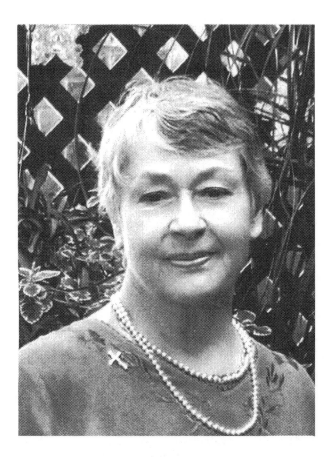

In Loving Memory
of
Nancy Coston

June 2, 1941 - June 11, 2013
Photo taken at 50th Anniversary - 2010

Introduction

This is what my wife Nancy and I learned over the period of 8 years while Nancy fought terminal disease.

The information is set up to be reviewed in multiple sessions. If you try to cover it all at once it can be overwhelming. Start with an initial review of about an hour. That step is to introduce the materials. Take your time. Perhaps use a highlighter. Trying to do too much at once would be very difficult and not a good idea. Do what you can manage and then revisit. Celebrate each accomplishment … no matter how small.

Approximately 50% of the US population will die of cancer or heart related disease. This write-up, although using cancer as the start point, can be used by many terminal patients, care givers, and families for the final journey that is ahead. The odds are that you do not have a very good idea of what you will have to go through. Nancy, and I had very little information about what we could have done to have made the journey easier. I have said uncountable times "dear Lord, how did this happen?" Now I know some of the answers. These notes will share them with you.

Terminal illnesses will put you through the following processes in this order: denial, confusion, frustration, anger, awareness, sadness, acceptance and then moving forward. The goal of these

Nancy Notes is to help patients and family members manage the terminal illness journey to reach a position of comfort and peace.

Allow me to describe the final journey in terms of you and your loved one driving from Vladivostok, Russia (North East coast) down to Beijing, China and then across to Moscow, Russia. You have some maps you can't read. 90%+ of the people you attempt to talk to do not speak English. You start with a handful of rubles and American credit cards. How do you pay for fuel? Where do you spend the night? Wait until you attempt to order food. This is not a detailed instruction manual. It is set up to show you where some of the pot holes are and to let you learn from actual experiences. Use this information to get you and your loved ones to thinking and planning ahead. Now; relate that to your journey. Here we go.

As you review these materials, usually two types of personalities will appear. You will probably automatically default to concentrating on one of the following areas.

A) Problem solving personality
    Finance
    Legal
    Activity lists: 65 before and 40 after death
    Reports: CBC (complete blood count), intensive care
B) Comforting personality
    Hospital and hospice activities
    How to comfort the loved one
    Insure final preparation of the body is done with dignity.
    Final "let me go" comments
C) Both personalities
    Morphine and drug impacts

PRIMARY PROBLEM AREA: Total confusion.

Let's start with the money. The money coming in for you to pay bills with is primarily controlled by bureaucrats. I call this the "money pipe". For simplicities sake we will assume the money flow starts primarily at the federal level and flows downward through all the rest of the money in: $$ SOURCES listed below. These people are charged to manage the funds to get the biggest bang for the buck. This means "control". Lots of pieces of paper. OK?

> $$ SOURCES: Federal $>>>State $>>>County $>>>
> Local $>>>Insurance $>>>Charity $>>>Others

Money out ($$ USES) is consumed by the following entities for the patient's benefit. More pieces of paper. In addition to surviving the rigors of illness management, you will need to have some idea of how to tie the source of funds to paying your bills. It can be difficult - but it can be done. At times irritating, but doable.

$$ USES: Hospitals – Doctors (nerves, lungs, lymph, x-ray/scans, oncology/cancer, bacterial/sepsis, hospice, pain control, cardio, etc.) - Nurses - Specialists - Physical therapists - Legal - Burial - Cremation - Memorial - Flowers -Hospice - Ambulance - Soc. Sec. - Medicare - Medicaid – insurance-grief counseling, etc. These are nice people but many of them lack communication skills. Also, it is next to impossible to touch base with the ones you need at the moment you want or need them. They are very busy people.

All suffers I have reviewed the information with have gone through almost exactly the same thing: Lack of: (1) overall knowledge, (2) planning, (3) communications from the medical community and

(4) heavy morphine and drug impacts. A lot of information will be coming at you. Again. It is doable.

All I can do is introduce you to the final journey. There are a lot of people available to help you. This was on Nancy's key chain. GOD. Grant me the serenity to accept the things I cannot change, the courage to change the things I can, and the wisdom to know the difference. AMEN.

Some people that helped me put the Nancy Notes together follow. They are from one side of the country to the other. Vaughn, Don, Judy, Chris, Jim, Judy, Larry, Dale, Shelba, Ralph, Barry, Marie, Sherry, Andy, Susan, Sandy, Scott, Grey, Jane, and many more.

Contents

SECTION #1

(1) Subject: Terminal illness.

I will cover what we needed to do and what we should have done after Nancy's diagnosis of terminal cancer: treatments, emergency ward, drugs, intensive care, hospice and more. Neither of us was ready for what would happen. We were better prepared than most. I will cover our correct actions and our omissions. I am not a doctor or a lawyer. This only what we experienced. I hope the reader will find some items of value. Remember, all the survivor will have left are memories. Make them as pleasant as possible.

(2) Background: The story starts February 20, 2005.

We were waiting for the call from the cancer clinic. Nancy answered the phone. A stunned expression came over her face. Nancy said a bad word. She turned to me and asked if I would support her. I said "of course". She walked over. We hugged. She said "I love you". I told her "I love you". The diagnosis was terminal blood cancer. Nancy was given 24 to 36 months to live. Nancy said "it will be an interesting journey". She went through radiation and 7 1/2 years of three times a month of chemo. Nancy did not go down easily. I can't remember one gripe in the eight years. The doctors called her a walking miracle. They were unable to understand how she survived that long. Nancy said "prayer had a lot to do with it".

I am not trying to antagonize the atheist with the following information. If I do not enter it here, the reader will not understand Nancy. Months after her death I noticed some tabs sticking out of her Bible. These were the only verses tabbed. The text was underlined. Nancy did this during the period immediately after the stem cell transplant and the horrible follow-up chemo

I didn't know what Nancy was reading when she went to her "quiet place". It makes me feel sad that I was not there to share with Nancy what she was doing. You do not want your loved one to suffer by themselves. I had no clue. I was working in our home office at the other end of the house. This is before she found a church and asked me to attend with her. I had no idea Nancy had found "The Bible".

In order, here is what the tabs were. Atheist or not, I think everyone should read these and the surrounding verses. Nancy never reviewed these with me. She was a very private person. Pretty good pickings by someone not yet familiar with the Bible

1)* Romans 8:18. In the same way, the Spirit helps us in our weakness. We do not know what we ought to pray for, but the Spirit himself intercedes for us with groans that words cannot express.

2)* Romans 10:9. That you confess with your mouth, "Jesus is Lord"' and believe in your heart that God raised him from the dead, you will be saved.

3)* Thessalonians 5:19. Do not put out the Spirit's fire.

4)* 1 John 1:1 Test the spirits to see whether they are from God.

4)* 1 John 1:8. Whoever does not love does not know God, because God is love.

* All from The Holy Bible, New International Version. Copyright 1973, 1978, 1984. International Bible society.

(3) First things to do:

(3:a) Legal instructions and requirements: copies, locations, and understanding.

After you get over the shock, this is one of the first things you should do. Get a competent person to help you. The documents will probably be multiple pages. Go slow. Be careful. Get help. Understand what you are doing.

The hospital MAY be able to direct you for source documents. If you have a pastor, use him also. You will need copies at your primary and Intensive Care hospitals on file. Include a completed statement of what heroic measures are permitted and an exception statement of when the patient can be brought out of sleep to say goodbye and give final wishes, maybe a hug. Neither my best bud and his wife who died a year earlier or I were given this opportunity.

When Nancy and I started the legal process we did not have a clue about how to prepare for death. The only thing we had was a will. We always figured we would be taken out together in an automobile accident. Boom. End of that story. We did a lot of traveling. Obviously that was wrong. When Nancy went into intensive care, years after we wrote our wills, neither one of us thought about the following activities.

The "Five Wishes" document (as of 2013) is legal in District of Columbia and 38 states. The Five Wishes has many check off sections for you. We both checked off the following heroic statement: "I do not want life support treatment. If this has been started, I want it stopped". I had to enforce this for Nancy. The ER was getting ready to put an air pipe down her throat. It turned out to be unnecessary. Try these on-line: Printable Version of Five Wishes or agingwithdignity.org.

The cover page of the Five Wishes shows the following: It is a multiple page document.

A) The Person I Want to Make Care Decisions for Me When I Can't
B) The Kind of Medical Treatment I Want or Don't Want
C) How comfortable I Want to Be
D) How I Want People to Treat Me
E) What I Want My Loved Ones to Know

2) Department of Veterans Affairs has a "Durable Power of Attorney for Health Care and Living Will".
3) Most states have their own documents.

* Try aarp.org and search "advance directive". Section #1

Exception Statements samples:

My opinion is that you should show these following two statements to ALL your supporting medical staff including doctors. Nancy and I wrote these ourselves.

a) Should a situation arise where my health care agent(s) feel I would like to have input on a situation or decision, I would like pain medicine reduced as needed, so that I can be alert. Nancy wrote and added this one herself.
b) If I am under heavy medication that makes me unable to communicate, and death is positive, ask my care giver if it would be time to bring me back to where I can say my last goodbye. This is the one we did not do. I wrote this up after her death.

I have never seen these two requests in a standard form. Again, I am not a lawyer or doctor. I was in such a turmoil with Nancy I never even thought about these. No one mentioned these options to me and Nancy. I have added them to my Five Wishes. Send copies to your kids/concerned adults.

You may have to get the medical attendants to bring your spouse back to where you can say finals. The doctors are not always there. You will need to tell medical personnel to do this. They will know if and when it can be done. The spouse will tell you if it is too uncomfortable. You both need this option. Bring your statements to the hospital if they are not already on file. The Docs and many medical people can come very close to telling when the end is near. You and your spouse should know what can happen after admittance. Most medical team's jobs are to keep the patient alive. Sometimes you come in second place. I believe Nancy's passing could have been easier (on me too).

Nancy was experiencing delirium from 3:30 PM (when she awoke from her nap Saturday at home) and never quite came back to mental clarity for the complete 11 days she spent in the hospitals. She was correctly kept doped up 100% of the time.

Read the Hospital/Critical Care DR's DAILY NOTES. (See Section #2) You generate questions from these. This is a great way to keep track of what is happening. Health providers are all nice people, but they communicate at a different level.

We could have discussed her going into Christ's waiting arms in her eternal heaven. We could have talked about me joining her. Planning ahead and being able to talk could have reduced vast amounts of highly visible confusion and frustration on her part. I am unable to express how upset she was. She could not express herself. She could not talk. Once she got into the hospital I didn't know if I should have mentioned her actual upcoming death to her. With foreknowledge I would have known how to comfort her. A final lucid I love you, a kiss and hug would have been nice.

(3:b) Bucket list Completed

I had a feeling Nancy was in serious trouble in March/April 2013. She went to God June 11, 2013. My plan was to finish what you will read next before she died. I did not get it completed. I had hoped to spend bunches of good times reviewing this with her in the Rocky Mountains during our annual trip to see family and celebrate the Fourth of July. Do not take your loved ones remaining time on this earth for granted. You may think you have ten years or more. Write it down. Speak to them now.

In ICU (intensive care unit) Nancy was extremely confused, angry and frustrated. One time when she came half way around for a minute she said "all I do is sleep and drink water". Later she said "I am so tired and weak. When she drank water she could only guide the straw. I had to hold up the weight of the cup. She could not talk, only point. We will talk about pain killers and morphine later. What we are covering at this point shows why the bucket list is required.

If you don't tell them how much you appreciate them while they are alive, I guarantee you can't tell them after death. I started this letter in mid-April 2013. I read it to Nancy completely 3 or 4 times during her hospital stay. She was very groggy, but I think she got all of it. I sure hope so. Get your "bucket list" done early. Mine was not finished. I know Nancy would have liked to have left me with a few comments also. We never thought about final words. Why should we? We had plenty of time until time ran out.

I failed to tell her that she was totally responsible for the success of our marriage.

The following is the first part of what I read to the church congregation at Nancy's memorial. Hopefully you can use this to get you started on your own list. Most of the hospital information will be in Section #2.

> This is a celebration of a giving life. Most of you didn't realize Nancy has been a walking miracle for the last 6 years, according to her Oncologist. She was diagnosed with multiple myeloma (terminal blood cancer) February 2005 at stage 3. When Nancy found our Church in 2008 her energy level was already down to 60 %. She wanted to do more with the church but was unable. By 3 months ago it was down to less than 40 %. I wish you had known her at 100 percent. Lots of people have asked, so I'll cover the medical summary after this Bucket List.
>
> Dear Nancy/Bitty
>
> The years we have spent together have been good. There have been rough spots, but so what? Without you I doubt I would have had a life. Literally. I would have probably killed myself drunk in an auto wreck. I would have had no education. Would not have learned enough to where I feel comfortable to talk with most anyone. Doubt I would have had any children. Much less ones that had any brains or character. You did a super job of raising them. That is an unbelievable gift to give someone. Thank you.
>
> There times I can look back and see you very clearly. In high school. At A&P. First date. Walking together in the woods. Bowling. (Then I mentioned a personal item or two).

Many of your girlfriends and acquaintances have come to me over the years and said "Nancy is absolutely beautiful". Women do not do that very often. I truly think you are still unaware of your beautiful features. (She shook her head "no" when I read this part. Nancy was unable to speak at that point.) You are totally unpretentious and unassuming. We have attended Gourmet clubs, Officer's club functions, bridge club, etc. We would go in with you all duded up with earrings, white sheath dresses, necklaces. You at 5 10 ½. You brought conversations to a halt. Then you would smile. Everything was cool. They all liked Nancy.

You took responsibility for raising the kids, gave me a home to come home to, backed me up every time I was not there - taking care of my crummy old cars, jobs, Navy, moving 16 times, meeting new neighbors, and setting up new houses. Then you always worked and worked without me even needing to ask for help. You were my traveling buddy. Fun to be with. We share our memories from High School till today. No one else can ever do that with me. Even the kids don't know what we are talking about.

You reintroduced me to my religion. Introduced me to a type of people I could not imagine. Some people call them Christians. Our pastor deserves vast amounts of credit. I have told you this before: you have been the love of my life, you are the love of my life and you will be the love of my life. No one can replace bitty.

I don't want to lose you, temporary as it will be. Thank you again.

Love, Jim (The above is what I read to her while she was in intensive care)

(3:b) Bucket list Not completed

I didn't get the list completed. It was to be finished in the three weeks prior to when we were going to the mountains for 4th of July celebration. Too little. Too late. This would have been a very small part of what I wanted to tell her. Allow me to summarize: Nancy was shy, reserved, stubborn, loving, giving, beautiful, unselfish and delightful. She was the most giving person I have ever known. These words may help the reader get started. Nancy had what is referred to in the Bible as a "servant's heart".

(1) There was never any time during our marriage that we were not under the gun. Continual pressure. At first financial, then her raising the children, then many moves, then developing a new company together, then eight years of fighting cancer. I just accepted her willingness to keep going with no complaints. I should have given her a lot more atta-boys

(2) There were times I was too demanding. I told a truly beautiful woman that she too heavy and unattractive and I avoided her. I had too much pride. Then I got angry. Then I got bitter and now I am sorry beyond words. This meant that my wants had not been satisfied. That had to hurt her tremendously. She never said a word. Some people, me included, will consider this a form of domestic abuse. Think about this? Have you done anything of this nature? What are you going to do about it?

The following is some knowledge I got from the Bible months after her death. One of the greatest pains in life is the pain of rejection. She may have gained the weight possibly because of the pressure I put her under. I think it may have been my fault. Nancy never voiced one word of complaint. When you marry a model you get spoiled. I demanded too much.

(3) I was also gone years for weeks at a time working. Actually more than a twenty year career in the military would demand. This was more serious pressure. Again, she never said a word. Nancy just kept working. I always tell others not to do as I did, but do as I say: try not to travel. There were other jobs I could have had. The dollars continued to beckon. I put too much of a load on her. I never apologized. Never thought about it.

(4) Dear Nancy I am so sorry I never asked you for forgiveness for the stupid, prideful things I did and the pressure I put you under.

In order, the most important things you gave me were 1) brought me to The Church, 2) gave your life and love to me and 3) gave me three wonderful children. I didn't completely realize these things until almost one year after her death. When she was with me I never thought about it. I took these things for granted.

The Lord just took her too quickly. I was too selfish, prideful and slow to react. Her life and the end could have been easier and better. At the end the joy of the Lord was her strength. Mine too. God will give you the strength to get through. It will be unbelievably difficult. I remember Nancy with love and gratitude. Not having been able to share this more with Nancy makes me feel incredibly guilty. You better address this before it is too late. Many I have talked to feel the same.

(3:c) Final overview:

Our pastor and I spent time going over the above and the medical activities weeks after the memorial and burial. I told him that "In 8 days in intensive care and 3 days in hospice I never had an opportunity to say good-by to Nancy nor her to me. No one told me that she could die until the 6th day". The Pastor's face collapsed at this point. To summarize - these were days of total confusion, first for Nancy and next for me.

I truly think these following paragraphs could be the most important ones in this presentation.

Early on define how you both enjoy talking about your life together. Some look back, some concentrate on today and some look to the future. I believe you will find that the closer people get to the life's end that they concentrate more on "today". Toward the end Nancy was 3% concerned about the past. Not keen on "remember when". She would discuss the kids. Her focus was 94% this week and next week. 3% futures. Put your interest in the background. Concentrate on what your spouse would find interesting. The conversation is not for you anymore.

During the total 11 days in ICU and hospice we never got the opportunity to say "remember when"…our first kiss, the first time we professed love for each other, our first little apartment, the time she cooked her first biscuits, (what a mess) running stoplights on the way to the hospital for our first child, Navy, travel, vacations, watching the children grow up to become really great people. None of the above. I have no idea what Nancy would have liked to talk about. She never mentioned whether she felt she had had a productive, enjoyable and satisfactory life.

To this day I do not know if she was ready to go "home in Heaven". It happened so fast. We had never discussed the actual circumstances of the physical death of either one of us. I found out later she would have liked to have spent her final days in our home as opposed to the hospice care unit. Nothing to it. Easily done. The drugs and our own failures to discuss these items much earlier removed all possibilities of talking about them after hospital admittance.

We did not know when to ask for spiritual support. Nancy's brother had been a pastor for 35 years. Our church pastor had been a friend for 19 years. We had two other retired pastors as church members. I used to have coffee with them at least once a week. All we had to do was ask. We could have discussed her going into Christ's waiting arms. How she would go home to her eternal heaven. We could have talked about me joining her. This could have reduced vast amounts of very obvious confusion, frustration, anger and perhaps fear. Once she got into the hospital I didn't know if I should mention her actual upcoming death to her. With foreknowledge I would have known how to approach and comfort her. Will she be able to have coffee with her parents, my mom and my aunt and uncle in Heaven? Again, I think a final lucid I love you, a kiss and hug would have been nice.

Sometime in mid-April 2013 we had just signed off on the purchase of our memorial headstone and were wondering what to do with our cremation ashes. Nancy said "Hobby Lobby will have something of use. Let's go." She picked a composite, old fashioned, two story house with dual gables to put her ashes in. She told me to paint the body cream and the roof brown. I did that plus put white paper curtains in the top floor and Christmas colored paper curtains on the bottom floor. I am going to use a mailing tube for myself. I have already painted it black. It has "Dad" on the lid/top in gold letters.

July 5th 2013 I placed her in her old fashioned "little house" prior to the burial memorial. She never got a chance to see it. Should I have tried to show it to her while she was in the ICU? The kids said "no". They told me she had known I would take care of it. It was neat. I wish she could have seen it.

We held the burial memorial in the Rocky Mountains. This was for family. They came from all over. Nancy is buried in our beautiful plot that we picked out in 2011 in the local cemetery at the top of a hill at about 9600 feet elevation looking out to the Santa de Christo Mountains. It is truly beautiful. Nancy liked it. She can also look the other way and watch the gold mining activities. Nancy liked the big trucks.

(4) Medical reports

(4:a) Oncologist/doctor's reports

Make sure you get copies of ALL Doctor's reports and transcripts prior to hospitalization. This could cover years - hopefully. Lots of valuable info there. The doctor's reports and CBC reports are the ones I made the most use of prior to Nancy going into intensive care. Set yourself up a 2 inch binder. Put in monthly tabs. When information comes in, just file it in date order. Set up separate files/ folders for insurance billing, payments and general information.

The following are some <u>very, very limited and simple</u> definitions. I got these on-line. The Docs will fill in the details. You will add and subtract from this list while building your own spread sheet(s) to track progress. Don't panic. You can do this. If you are not into spreadsheets, ask someone that likes this kind of stuff to help you. As a last resort you can use the old fashioned manual "green ledger accounting sheets". Remember the basic condition driving the information shown is cancer. Heart disease and diabetes would probably fit also.

Everyone is different. You should build your own data sheets when you start your journey. Between you and your specialist you will be able to pick out the most important values to track.

WBC   "white blood cell" Fights infection.
RBC   "red blood cell" Carries oxygen.
HGB   "hemoglobin" Oxygen carrying pigment in the red blood cell.
HCT   "hematocrit" % of RBC's in whole blood.
PLT   "platelets" Help clot the blood.
MVP   "mean platelet volume" average volume or size of platelets.
MCV   "mean corpuscular volume" average volume or size of a RBC
MCH   "mean corpuscular hemoglobin" average weight of HGB of each RBC.
MCHC "mean corpuscular hemoglobin concentration in the average RBC.
Anemia is defined as a lack of the proper amount of blood cells.

The first treatment Nancy had was radiation to kill the bone infection area. This occurred In March. First a series of x-rays were performed to locate the damaged areas. Multiple myeloma eats bone. This shows on x-rays. Then the focused radiation procedures take place. This killed the severely infected bone damaged areas. Then meds/chemicals are given to strengthen and regrow the damaged bone(s). This provides a foundation for the muscles to attach to. When we started we did not know enough at that time to keep complete medical reports. We figured this out pretty quickly. Examples follow for you to use.

All health problems are different. This spreadsheet was Nancy's. I ran it for eight years starting 3/08/2005. We took it with us to every doctor appointment. I think most standard hospital reports will get you into the detail so deeply you cannot tell where you are. Even some of our doctors made use of this format.

The first report that follows is an example of Nancy's oncologist's reports. Remember, there are lots of different involved doctors. Get your reports from all of them. The second report is the CBC report. It is the source for the spread sheet example that follows. There is another set of reports. They were generated while Nancy was in the hospital ICU. The ones I show you here were called Intensive Care Doctor's Dictation. This information stands on its own and will be covered in Section #2. Examples will be included.

HEMATOLOGY AND ONCOLOGY DIAGNOSIS: Multiple myeloma and patient has now developed myelodysplastic syndrome either spontaneously or from melphalan from her bone marrow transplant or Revlimid that she was on; it is hard to say. She has a plethora of cytogenetic changes which would give this an adverse overall prognosis, so I think prognosis may not be so good right now. She is stable. We could use Vidaza and Dacogen only when she becomes high-grade and transfusion dependent. Prior to that time, we would of course, give her Erythropoietin/Aranesp a chance.

We did a workup with folate, B12, TSH, retic counts, parvovirus, a very complete workup in terms of other etiologies but bone marrow biopsy definitely sees that this is MDS. She had an IgA and multiple myeloma with standard risk features diagnosed in 2005. Seven years ago she was on thalidomide and dexamethasone by my previous partner, Dr. Delgalvis. She had a bone marrow transplant. Two months after the transplant her disease started worsening and she was on Velcade for 8 cycles. She had a lot of toxicity and peripheral neuropathy and then counts started to escalate. Later on, years after she had the 8 cycles of Velcade, she was put on low dose Revlimid and dexamethasone. We stopped her Revlimid and dexamethasone. Her counts continued to decrease. She gets very short of breath and it turned out that she was dropping her hemoglobin and hematocrit on all of her counts. We did a bone marrow biopsy and her myeloma is behaving, but unfortunately now has a diagnosis of myelodysplastic syndrome.

MEDICATIONS: She is on albuterol, calcium, Aleve, Lyrica, Ambien, aspirin, acyclovir and Pepcid.

REVIEW OF SYSTEMS: Except for the shortness of breath, she feels pretty good. She can walk. She can exercise. There has been no fever or chills, no infection. She feels a little swollen, which she is, a little bit fatigued and some memory and concentration

CBC with Diff Protocol

Results
Abnormal

Status: **Final result**
10/11/2012 8:51 AM

6a) 2

Entry Data
10/11/2012

Component Results

Component	Value	Flag	Reference Range	Status
WBC	2.7	L	4.0-10.7 K/UL	Final
RBC	2.06	L	3.8-5.5 M/UL	Final
HGB	6.1	L	11.7-15.6 G/DL	Final
HCT	23.3	L	34.2-46.0 %	Final
MCV	113	H	80-99 FL	Final
MCH	35.0	H	27-33 pg	Final
MCHC	34.6		32-36 G/DL	Final
Platelet Count	47	L	130-400 K/UL	Final
RDWCV	20.4	H	10.0-15.5 %	Final
MPV	9.5		7.4-11.0 FL	Final
Seg Neutrophils	39	L	43-75 %	Final
Lymphocytes	49	H	15-40 %	Final
Monocytes	10		3-12 %	Final
Eosinophils	2		0-3 %	Final
Neutrophils, Absolute	1.05	L	1.9-7.0 K/UL	Final
Lymphocytes, Absolute	1.33		1.0-4.8 K/UL	Final
Monocytes, Absolute	0.27		0.0-0.8 K/UL	Final
Eosinophils, Absolute	0.05		0.0-0.45 K/UL	Final
Diff Type	AUTO			Final

Lab and Collection
CBC with Diff Protocol (⬛⬛⬛⬛⬛⬛⬛⬛ on 10/11/12 - Lab and Collection Information

Result History
CBC with Diff Protocol ⬛⬛⬛⬛⬛⬛⬛⬛ on 10/11/12 - Order Result History Report

CBC with Diff Protocol
[500195]
Lab

Authorizing: ⬛⬛⬛⬛⬛⬛⬛,
DO
Department: ⬛⬛⬛⬛⬛⬛⬛

Date: 10/11/2012
Released ⬛⬛⬛⬛⬛⬛⬛
By: ⬛

Order Mode

Action	Order Mode	Communicator	Responsible Provider	Signed By	Signed On
Ordering	Transcribed	⬛⬛⬛⬛		Signature Not Required	

Original Order

Ordered On	Ordered By
Thu Oct 11, 2012 8:06 AM	⬛⬛⬛⬛⬛⬛⬛

Reprint Requisition
CBC with Diff Protocol ⬛⬛⬛⬛⬛⬛⬛ on 10/11/12

Order Questions

Question	Answer	Comment

(4:b) CBC Spread Sheet

The primary blood cell levels we tracked were: WBC white, RBC red, HGB hemoglobin, PLT platelets. Cancer indicators were IGA and lamda light chains. Your doctor can give you definitions and impacts. Your job is to follow the changes. Note the trend of changes in the blood cells.

Date	WBC	RBC	HGB	PLT	HCT	BUN	ALB	TP	IGA	SGOT	SGPT	CREAT	LAMDA
10/18/2011	3.1	3.29	12.10	92	35.8	13	3.3	6	254	21	19		
11/10/2011	3.5	3.05	11.10	100	33.1	13	3.5	6.1			19		1.62
12/22/2011	4	3.31	12.40	70	35.9	17	3.5	5.1	208	14	20		
1/19/2012	4	3.32	12.30	68	36.2	17	3.6	5.1					
2/23/2012	3.2	3.32	12.50	91	36.2	14	3.4	6.2	225	18	19		
4/18/2012	3.2	3.39	13.00	85	37.2	15	3.7	6.7	225	19	19		1.52
7/10/2012	3.6	3.06	11.50	71	33.2	18	3.5	6.2	216	15	19		1.49
Last Revlimid 7/26/2012													
8/14/2012	3.4	2.64	9.10	53	26.7		4.4	6.4	249	17	26		1.49
9/20/2012	2.7	2.06	8.10	47	23.3	17	3.5	5.9		17	26	0.8	1.53
10/11/2012 (Transfusion 10/12 - Bone Marrow Biopsy 10/11)	2.7	2.87	10.40	55	30.9	16	3.8	6.4		20	27		
10/22/2012	3.4	2.87	10.90	65	31.5				244			0.7	1.69
11/5/2012	3.8	2.85	10.20	57	30.3	18	3.9	6.1	250	24	32	0.8	1.40
12/13/2012	3.9	2.63	10.50	47	30.3	14	3.7		213		33	0.9	
1/17/2012	3.3	2.49	9.60	48	28.8		3.7		222	18		0.8	1.33
2/12/2012	2.1	2.48	9.50	44	28.7		Aranesp Injection #1(300mg)						
2/25/2013	3	2.30	9.00	46	26.4		Aranesp Injection #2 (300mg)						
3/18/2013	2.1	1.88	7.30	46	21.4	13	3.4	5.5	Aranesp Injection #3 (500mg)				
4/1/2013	2.1	2.61	9.20	44	27.2				218	19	27	Transfusion - 2bags	
4/8/2013						21.3 Aranesp Injection #4 (500mg)							

Date	WBC	RBC	HGB	PLT	HCT	BUN	ALB	TP	IGA	SGOT	SGPT	CREAT	LAMDA
4/18/2013	2.5	2.49	8.70	52	26.8						Transfusion - 2bags		
4/29/2013	2.1	2.02	7.30	61									
5/14/2013	2.9	2.23	7.90	79	23.1		Transfusion - 2 bags						
5/15/2013						Port installed							
5/22/2013	2.9	2.96	9.60	75	29.5	Last transfusion. No help.							
5/29/2013													
5/30/2013													

Autologous Stem Cell Transplant, August 2005

This was the next step in Nancy's battle with cancer after radiation. You will need all sorts of telephone numbers to keep track of what is happening and what is going to happen, including travel. This procedure took almost two months. The process involves removing the blood, running it through a centrifuge to remove as many stem cells as possible for later use, freezing them, doing chemo to try to kill the cancer cells remaining in the body, then putting the stem cells back in and staying at a "clean" hotel for a month, going back to the hospital every day to insure you have not come down with infections (at this stage you start with having no white cells to fight infection). The odds of survival for this procedure were in the high 97% plus range. When the nurses were putting the stem cells back in Nancy they said she was starting her life all over again. I remember sitting there with them. After all this, in three weeks the process failed. The cancer came back with a vengeance. That was the only time I saw Nancy get mad and cry. Then she had to start on heavy dose chemo again three times per month for the next 7 1/2 years. I was numb. Nancy handled it better than I did.

Doctors-Autologous Transplant

AUTOLOGOUS TRANSPLANT	Start planning end of May
Mark	1-800
Stacy transplant coordinator	1-800
Teri Training & support	1-800
Judy Clinic coordinator	999-
Jim	999-
Nancy	999-
Scott	@l.com

St front desk   (700-
Insurance Co. Dr. OK on $ PPO   1-800 ext
Customer Service   1-800

Re-evaluate/restage
X-rays, CAT, blood work (4 days) Home   6/27-6/30

Start process   City   7/5 – 7/7
Catheter insert @ hosp.

Stay @ the xxx @   City

7:00 7/6   Review and consent
8:30 7/6   Psychological review and learn about how to maintain
           catheter.
8:00 7/7   Line flush class for care givers (this will probably
           be you)

Mobilization (priming)   (9 days)   Home   7/11-7/19
Prep for Cytoxan – 5 hours
CTX Cytoxan one infusion. – 3 ½ hours Kills cancer cells
           Insure liver and bladder is flushed. Too much water.
           Emergency!!!!
           Increase white cells. Neupogen (11 days all the way
           through City)

1:00 Last day mobilization   (1 day)   City   7/20
                               Stay @ xxx

Stem cell collection (harvest) (2 days)   City   7/21-7/23
           6+ hours per day – hospital
           4.2 volume total collection. Enough for only one transplant.

Pre-transplant education class	@ 4:00 PM City (Care giver - Pop)		7/26
Vacation/recuperate	(4 days)	Las Vegas	7/27

AUGUST
Hi-dose chemo Melflin

Kill cancer cells	(1 - days)	City	8/1-8/3
Re-infusion stem cells	(1 - days)	City	8/4

Inn	(4 weeks)	City	8/5

Recovery (24 hour surveillance)

Scott	8/8
Pop	8/13
Sandy	8/18
Pop	8/24 to 8/30

University of AAAA	Second opinion. No help. $25,000.

(5) Change of subject. Notes for old folks.

June 6 or 7. 2:00 PM in ICU. Nancy's brother and his wife and I were talking and I said "what about this idea?" After a certain point of marriage (40 years +?) your love for your spouse not only gets stronger but it changes. It is deeper, more familiar, more comfortable, and better. Our last 8 years were like that. What a blessing. Perhaps Nancy's diagnosis of terminal cancer shocked us into reaching that point. I don't know. I believe I saw the same thing in Nancy. We didn't even know enough to talk about it. Not only did they feel this to be true, but other "old folks" I have reviewed this with feel the same way. Look for it.

For example: You enjoy doing the same old things again and again. Going to the same grocery store multiple times per week, driving 1600 miles one way to see the kids again and again, looking for the same old Denny's. You name it. We had fun. It really hurts when it ends. The survivor pays dearly for that level of love and comfort. But, without those years how would you attain that level and been able to share and enjoy it? I wish someone had told us about this years ago. Then we would have made a conscious effort to enjoy our final years together even more. We didn't know enough to recognize the change and talk about it. What a loss. We were more comfortable with each other but did not know why. Maybe we didn't really grow up until Nancy was diagnosed. She sure gave me a lot. She is my girl forever. Never got to tell her this.

Something for the kids

The church memorial was held in our local church. The burial memorial was held in the Rocky Mountains hundreds of miles from our home. I got so buggered up getting all the arrangements made that I misplaced this piece of paper. The root of this took place in 1963 when I refused to get the kids started in church after Nancy asked me to. It cut into my Sunday morning sleep. Worst decision I ever made. It was 45 years later when Nancy found a church for us. The following is what I wanted to tell them. Maybe the reader can use this. Here goes.

10:00 AM Burial memorial. July 5, 2013. This burial memorial for Mom may be the last chance I will ever have all of you together. What I am going to say is for Sherry, Scott, Sandy and their children. Is there anything you would give up your life for, right now, today? Think about that. There is something that I would do this for.

You are aware that your mom was a Christian woman of great faith. Perhaps God took her in order that I could tell you this. Mom was a giving person. This may be the last thing she gives to us. If any or all of you could sometime during your life attain her level of Christian faith, I would be more than willing to give my life up for you.

You will not be walking down the street and be struck by the "faith lightning bolt". It takes time. It is up to you. God provides us with an independent will. After much study with qualified help, you can make up your mind. Right now none of you know enough to make an informed decision.

You choose belief - yes or no. There is no perhaps. I can get you started. Also, you may not ever have access to your pastor uncle, like this again. It is up to you.

Notes for Christians (and others if curious)

The following is what I remember from a number of TV Pastors, Professors and PHD psychologist types instructing people about losing loved ones: Most were not over their losses. They all said to prepare for suffering. Physical, mental and emotional. This section is a bit of a downer, but I thought they had good points. I will attempt to summarize what was said.

(1) Prior to death. Expect to suffer. Identify actions to reduce the loneliness and possible depression.

Remember:
Jesus suffered for you.
You both must learn and grow during the process.
Nancy called it her "journey".

After loss: Loved one is in Heaven in God's arms
You will be joined again. Coffee time.
Tell them you love them. Many times. Words are good.

(2) During the final journey. Work on reducing the suffering.

Don't just sit there and let it happen. Work on these "Nancy Notes"
That is what I call them. Sitting there causes you emotionally go
down and get depressed. Do something. Plan, share, comfort and
do more than is required. Communicate and together stay on top
of what is happening. This will help your emotions stay up. Tell
them "I got you covered".

(3) After death for the survivor. See activity list.

The goal is to have less negative carryover after your loss. Go up,
not down. This is just one of many stories of this nature I could tell
you. A man's wife of many years died. He went into hibernation
for two solid years. Sat in his house all by himself. He almost died.
Very fortunately he found a lady to be a companion and later on
his wife. I'm not saying get married. The point is that you could
have some tough times ahead without your spouse.

Philippians 3:13-14.	Do not brood on the past - move ahead.
Matthew 6:27.	If you worry, can you add a single hour to your life?
Matthew 6:34	Don't worry about tomorrow. Tomorrow will take care of itself. Every day has enough problems of its own.
Matthew 6:9:13 (Lord's Prayer)	Our father who is in heaven, Holy is your name ....
Psalms 23: 4	Even though I walk through the valley of the shadow of death ....

The Lord is close to the brokenhearted. The reader of the Nancy Notes is not alone.

I guess all readers have heard someone say "why me"? The following may help get you started.

What can/will you learn from the process? Inward change. Growth.

How can/will you use your new found knowledge to help others? Outward change. Sharing.

> In summary: you can change for the better or for the bitter. What virtues can you develop?

** Keep your attitude positive. The two of you will have remembering to do - together - in the future.

Here is a book you need to buy. "Heaven. Your Real Home" by Joni Eareckson Tada. I have read it twice as of this writing. It helped me. It is referenced again in Section #2, 10:00 AM Wed. Yes 3 Times. I liked the following pages a bunch.

15, 23, 28-29, 35, 36, 44, 49, 58, 60, 70, 79, 85, 90, 100, 107, 110, 122, 127, 131, 137, 147, 150, 151, 157-158, 175, 180, 186, 190, 196-199, 201.

Here is another book I liked. "The Joshua Code" by O. S. Hawkins. Try the following pages.

93, 102, 105, 111, 129, 146, 147, 157, 173, 191-195, 206, 222, 227, 229, 237, 241-242, 263, 267.

Teach us to number our days carefully that we may develop wisdom in our hearts.

Value of small church groups. Join at least two of them.

Waiting on God = difficult. Your will be done.

Here are a few more "pastor" items. It will give you more benefits if you look them up as opposed to me feeding them to you.

> Isiah 41:10, Isiah 41:13, Psalm 52:8,
> Psalm 73:23-24, Psalm 119:28.

(6) Songs

We sang "Amazing Grace", her favorite song, at both memorials. Then I read "I Will Rise". Someone may like to use these. Nancy's second favorite song was "Wings Of A Dove". No one knew this one except Nancy. Ferlin Husky - 1960. You will need to look up the last two. Copyright laws make it too difficult for me to add them here.

Amazing Grace

Amazing grace how sweet the sound
That saved a wretch like me
I once was lost but now am found
Was blind but now I see

'Twas grace that taught my heart to fear
And grace my fears relieved
How precious did that grace appear
The hour I first believed

The Lord has promised good to me
His Word my hope secures
He will my shield and portion be
As long as life endures

Through many dangers toils and snares
I have already come
"Tis grace hath brought me safe thus far
And grace will lead me home

When we've been there ten thousand years
Bright shining as the sun
We've no less days to sing God's praise
Than when we first begun

Sample obituaries

I don't know what to tell you here. I knew things were going bad. I got us started by cutting examples from the newspaper for ideas for both of us. I figured that would make it easier on Nancy if I did mine also. You probably should do this as far ahead as possible. Nancy got the first paragraph written and then ran out of steam. The kids finished it after her death. I think they did a great job. I added a few sentences. I worked on mine just to provide support while Nancy was working on hers.

Nancy M Coston
June 2, 1941 – June 11, 2013

Nancy left this earth Tuesday, June 11, 2013, after battling cancer for eight years, walking hand in hand with Jesus to her eternal home. She is survived by her best friend, traveling buddy, love of her life, husband of 52 years, Jim Coston. Also her 3 devoted children, Sherry, Scott and Sandra, two sons-in-law, one daughter-in-law, and 6 adoring grandchildren.

- Nancy was born in Denver on June 2nd 1941, the 2nd child of Martha G. and Chester B. Miles. The Miles relocated to Birmingham, Alabama where Nancy met and married her high school sweetheart, Jim in 1960, and began their family. Nancy, Jim and the kids relocated numerous times, getting to see many great places. While living in North Carolina, Nancy graduated from Central Piedmont Community College, earning a degree in dental assisting. Best grades ever earned. Straight A's. Nancy also enjoyed being a member of her local bowling league. While living in Pennsylvania, they purchased an 1892 Victorian home which Nancy and Jim restored to its former glory with 1 ½ years of hard labor and love. They were members of a gourmet club and enjoyed many interesting dining experiences, some of which Jim would not eat. Nancy again joined a local bowling league. In 1994, Nancy and Jim settled in Grand Junction where they partnered together professionally and began their own tax and accounting business. While in Colorado, she was blessed to reconnect with her brother Don and sister-in-law Judy. The traveling buddies spent many great times exploring the West. Nancy enjoyed trying new recipes, gardening, reading, travel, crochet and politics. She could be described as one of the most unselfish, giving, unassuming people you could ever meet. She will be sorely missed and never forgotten.
- Nancy's family would like to thank friends, the local Church community, medical support team members for their love and prayers. The most wonderful wife and mother ever, we wish she could still be here! Jim is looking forward to enjoying her company for eternity in heaven.
- A memorial service and reception for Nancy will be held on Tuesday, June 25 at 11:00 am.

James M "Jim" Coston, Jr., born Birmingham, Alabama, July 18, 1940. Passed away on --------------- at some place. ----------------
Cause of death was ----------------

Jim was preceded in death by his wife, Nancy, his High School sweetheart and love of his life for 52+ years of marriage. Jim is looking forward to enjoying her company for eternity in heaven. His greatest accomplishment was their marriage and their three children. When discussing the kids he liked to introduce them as successful, functioning members of society.

Education: Four year BS in 30 months from Samford University. Worked as a salesman for State Farm Insurance, Co. during that time.

Military: Five years as Communications Officer, US Navy. Experienced the politics firsthand of the Viet Nam war. Was aware of when the North Viet Nam gun boats allegedly shot at our DD's in the Bay of Tonkin, and was the pre deployment communications and security inspections officer when the USS Pueblo was deployed to the area off North Korea after he had failed them in their inspections.

After that Jim and Nancy really started traveling. He worked in the following areas.

(1) Manufacturing (industrial engineer, Foreman, Plant Super, Production Mgr responsible for 5 plants and 2000 employees, Operation Mgr w/P&L responsibility). As consultant developed the Manufacturing Concepts and Implementation methodology and manuals used worldwide for the UNISUS Corp. Justified, developed, taught, managed and implemented systems in some 80 facilities as far away as Yugoslavia.

(2) Owner of: MLS and BYS systems. Developed concepts, designed, developed every data element, all logic, reports and implementation methods for both Maintenance and Production systems.

MLS. Maintenance Logic System used by: Shaw Carpets, Hagendaz, Johnson & Johnson, Volkswagen and many others. MLS was used from South Korea to Australia to South America and across the US.

BYS incorporated: Contained both critical path and Short Interval Scheduling, order entry tied to capacity requirements planning at order promise point, bill of material processor with total pegging, inventory with automatic removal and replacement during MRP runs/reruns and shop floor reporting, backward and forward finite and infinite scheduling from order entry to suppliers all based on chaos logic. Worked like a charm.

(3) Owner Tax and Accounting Solutions: The last year before selling that business Nancy produced 700 W-2 and 1099 forms by herself and Jim turned out 120 tax returns. 84 of those were for businesses in Grand Junction, Co. They knew a lot of people.

He is survived by three super children, Sherry, Scott and Sandra, two sons-in-law, one daughter-in-law, and six wonderful grandchildren. Nancy and Jim are buried on a rise at 9600 feet elevation overlooking the Santa De Cristo Mountains.

SECTION #2

1) Nancy getting weaker
2) Into the hospital
3) Hospice Location
4) Hospice care
5) Lymphodema
6) Morphine
7) Early life style changes
8) Oximeter
9) Bereavement

(1) Nancy getting weaker

Mid July 2012 Phone call with Sherry. Nancy had told Sherry that the chemicals were changing her personality. They were making her mean. Sherry told me Nancy was getting snippy. Sandy told Sherry that Nancy would come in and rearrange her kitchen. Over the last year or so I had noticed she was getting more opinionated and a bit pushy. It was so gradual I didn't care. No problem. For a person with her giving personality it was bothering her greatly.

July 28, 2012 Last heavy chemo (Revelimid) for the multiple myeloma. Nancy's decision. She told her oncologist "it made her feel bad". I was sitting there with her. The Dr. said we can give it a try. Worked OK for a while. This may have been the break point. Wish I had known. See Lymphedema.

Sept 2012 Started getting more tired quicker. Next CBC scheduled for October11, 2012.

Oct 11, 2012 CBC came back bad. Got 2 bone marrow biopsies. A new type blood cancer was discovered. Multiple myeloma produces too few blood cells. The new one produces lots of immature white cells. Called myelodysplastic syndrome. Nancy's life expectancy was reduced to one to two years. She wanted to know. Black and white. Her oncologist had a hard time telling Nancy.

Oct 12, 2012 Transfusion. OK for 5 ½ months. Nancy still pretty tired.

Mar 15, 2013 At church Joanne noticed Nancy's face was looking puffy. The lymph system problems were showing greatly. Legs, tummy, arms, etc.

Apr 1, 2013 Transfusion. OK for one month. When transfusions need to be this close together it is a very bad sign.

Apr 8 - 11 Daughter Sherry and Karl, husband visited. We went to the desert with them. Nancy did not have enough energy to take a long walk. We walked about 30 yards and stood by while Karl and Sherry took a 600 yard trail. Nancy stood by again while I went with them on second 250 yard walk. She was afraid to try the hike as she as she had no energy and the steepness of the trail could give her severe problems.

Apr 30, 2013 Transfusion. OK for 2 weeks.

May 15, 2013 Transfusion, OK for 2 weeks.

I think the sepsis bacterial infection had started during this time. People that have compromised immune systems should not crawl around in a garden. I know this is where she picked up a bug. She complained about hitting and scratching her knee. It was inflamed and started swelling within days.

May 20, 2013 Daughter Sandy and Scott, husband come to visit.

May 22, 2013 Last set of CBC labs. Low blood count. Dr. schedules a port install and transfusion.

(2) Into the hospital

May 28, 1013 Nancy was slowly cleaning house. She wouldn't quit. While talking to Sandy that night Nancy said she did not know if she could face another round of chemo. Nancy told Sandy that during the first chemo she wanted to crawl into a hole and die. Prayer was a large part of her survival at that time. She was willing to consider one more chemo try. Sandy told Nancy that she and I acted like friends. Nancy looked at Sandy and told her "he is my best friend". Nancy had never told me that. She was a very private person. Sandy asked Nancy what I would do after she was gone. Nancy said "he can take care of himself". That was very true, but it has been very difficult on many levels. Talk to each other and family about this ahead of death.

I know the sepsis bacterial infection really started to accelerate during this time frame. Was infection in her knee the probable source?

A Few Definitions

athogen:	Anything that can cause a disease. Is an infectious agent. Soil contamination is one of the most persistent sources. **REMBER THIS.**
Bactereremia:	Bacteria in the blood. Can cause sepsis and septic shock which has a relatively high mortality rate. Treatment is antibiotics.
Neutropenic sepsis:	Lack of white cells. Can bring on confusion. See June 1 following.
Pseudomonas infection (sepeticemia):	From common bacteria. Common in soil, water, plants, hospitals. Has high antibiotic resistance. Chemo patients are at high risk. Will attack a compromised immune system. Can result in high fever, chills, confusion and shock.
Dyspnea:	Hard to breath. Airway disease.
Tachypnea:	Rapid breathing > 20 breaths per minute. Puffing. Nancy got up to about 70 at the end.

Edema:	Liquid accumulation anywhere. Swelling. Minor =1, moderate =2, heavy =3
Pulmonary edema:	Liquid in lungs.
Erythema:	Infection causing capillaries to dilate.
Pseudomonas:	Infection caused by a common bacteria
Metastasize:	See doctor
Cancer stages:	Too many variables for this paper. See your doctor.
PTA:	Prior to admittance
DNR:	Do not resituate
SOB:	Shortness of breath
COPD:	Chronic obstructive pulmonary disease
Neuropathy	Healthy nerves do not burn

Into the hospital

May 29, 2013 Wed. @ 6:30 AM. Go to hospital for port installation. 7:30 AM Sandy and Scott depart to Atlanta. Afterward Nancy was feeling droopy. Her knee was hurting.

May 30, 3013 Thur. 8:00 AM transfusion. Did not have the usual boost. Should have read Nancy Notes Bucket List to her then.

May 31, 3013 Fri. Nancy's knee was really inflamed; swollen, hot and discolored. It hurt. We saw a Dr. at 10:30AM. Next we picked up the prescribed antibiotic. I feel as though we should have gone to the emergency ward at that point. Home at noon. It was hard for her to breathe. Then she developed the shakes. I should have taken her to the emergency ward then. Nancy was shaking so badly she had a hard time holding her cup up to take the antibiotics. I had to help her hold the cup. When someone is anemic or being hit with infection they can go hot or cold in a flash. What are you supposed to do? What do you look for? Talk to your doctor about this months ahead of time. Ask your doctor to read this section with you. I hope you do not need this information. Do not take a chance. Learn the signs and have the doctor tell you exactly what to do. I covered her with a heating pad and blanket. 30 minutes later she quit shaking. She went to bed and to sleep at 5:30 PM. Bad things were happening to Nancy. I missed the clues.

June 1, 2013 Sat. Nancy woke up at 6:00 AM. I do not remember what happened during the morning. She went back to sleep from 1:00 to 3:30 PM. She awoke disoriented and very weak. To me it looked like oxygen deprivation. See Neutropenia sepsis: The lack of white cells can bring on confusion. I would ask her a question and she could get only 4 to 5 words out and would then grind to a halt. Her knee really hurt. 4:30 PM. I helped Nancy with her walker into our car. We went to the emergency ward. I had to use a wheel chair to get her out of the car. Nancy was continuing to have breathing problems. In the emergency ward the doctor was not happy with Nancy's condition. Her knee and port were very, very swollen and inflamed. This was awful. The doctor said she could crash/die within minutes. No ventilator was permitted via legal wishes that were on file with the hospital. I never got to clearly speak to her after that. Nancy did say "do not bring the kids". Nancy fully planned on going home. You may want to look into your spouse's eyes and show and express love at this time. You may not get another chance. Nancy was disoriented.

Admission Information June 1, Saturday PM Doctor's Notes

Nancy M Coston is a 71yr old female who has been admitted with a chief complaint of progressive weakness and dyspnea over 4 days. Now presenting with fever, and concerns for bacteremia, early sepsis. (I think she was beyond early. JMC)

She had a port put in 4 days ago with declining IV access and received a RBC transfusion. She felt no improvement in dyspnea and energy with that, and 2 days later developed a tender red indurated patch over her left patella. Saw a DR. on Friday who found no fluid collection to tap, and started her on Keflex. However, over last two days she has noted new tender red blotches over the neck and right arm, and felt increasingly weak, more dyspnea and intermittently confused. Her home SATS dropped from usual 95% RA to 85-88%. Today feverish and worsening weakness, dyspnea, she presented to the ER with her husband.

PHYSICAL EXAM: Upon admittance to Emergency Room. General appearance - alert, pale, ill, but nontoxic appearing,

Mental status - alert, oriented to person, place, and time, normal mood, behavior, speech, dress, motor activity, and thought processes. (This was her last very lucid period. It lasted about thirty minutes. JMC)

Sunday 6/2/2013 (Next morning. Nancy's 72nd Birthday)

Intensive care DR's notes - summaries

The following are parts of summaries of some 80 ICU Doctor reports available to me/you.

HISTORY OF PRESENT ILLNESS: The **patient is a delightful** 72-year-old woman who was admitted 1 day ago with an infected vascular port. The port had been recently placed. There is redness and swelling around the port. She has multiple myeloma and myelodysplasia syndrome and requires frequent transfusions.

Risks.

She understands these can be life threatening complications of her myeloma; is a bit scared, nervous. She and her husband still feel DNR is most appropriate in her situation. (Nancy was very strong. JMC) Biopsy discussed with patient, and she agrees to anything that could help lead to answer / make her better. (No one told me about this later discussion with Nancy. JMC)

June 2, 2013 Sun. Removed the port. There was very heavy, visible bacterial infection at this time. Started the custom antibiotics, (4 different cocktails, each lasted 2 hours, then the procedure would be repeated) plus morphine and oxygen. Never got to the point to where she was even 20% clear- headed for 2 minutes. I never saw the CBC reports from this point forward. Never thought to ask for them. After 8 years I had a good understanding of CBCs. The Drs. were doing what they were trained to do: keep Nancy alive. They took control of her life away from her. The best I could tell no options were provided at that time. They did their job. You will have to push for options. I gave Nancy her last birthday card.

June 3, 3013 Mon. CRT and MRI. One of the Docs came in and asked Nancy "who is that?" pointing at me. She was groggy and didn't say anything. He asked again. She said "husband." I liked that. That is a lot more important than "Jim". It meant more to me. The doctor also asked her what day it was. All she could do was point over his shoulder. The doctor did not look happy. He asked her again. She smiled and pointed again. She could not speak, but I could tell something was amusing her. Her eyes were smiling. He looked over his shoulder. Three feet away, on the wall behind him, was a great big day calendar. Nancy snookered the doctor. That's my girl. See what I have lost!

June 4, 2013 Tue. No one knew it yet (I think) but, the vascular system and pulmonary alveoli (sacs) were damaged beyond repair by this time. Nancy was able to tell me once "I am so weak and so tired. All I do is sleep and drink water". I mention this to give you a feel for what can happen. You need to be aware of this type occurrence and plan on how to react. Then, a friend came and sang Amazing Grace. Nancy told her that was her favorite song. (I was unable to hear Nancy tell her.) I didn't know that was her favorite song. She enjoyed the music. Nancy actually tapped her fingers in time to the music. Her brother and his wife were there. Amazing Grace and I Will Rise were sang and read at her church memorial. Her second favorite song was Wings Of A Dove.

Impacts of drugs.

There were tears in the congregation after I finished reading the following to them at her memorial.

June 5, 2013 Wed. Speaking through morphine, Nancy awoke around 1:30 AM and told me "I am going to die". She appeared afraid. Her eyes were glazed. Others I have talked to have experienced the same thing. Even under morphine she figured it out before I did and before the doctors told us. Nancy was not ready for this. She was incredibly upset. This was a complete surprise to her. She had been planning on going home. Nancy was already putting together the food for our upcoming trip to the mountains for the 4th of July. Her garden was going gangbusters. All the flowers she planted were coming up.

What should I have done that night? What should I have said? Nancy could not accept the claustrophobia of the O2 mask. That kept her even more upset. Around 2:00 AM I talked her into one more 12 hour period of hanging on. I thought she would live. Perhaps this was when we should have said final goodbyes. I never told her I will miss you. Nancy never got to say anything. There was so much left unsaid. She was experiencing great morphine delirium by that point. Nancy went through a period where she said the children were not mine. The invective continued. Later she said they were not hers. Something had made her so mad at me she would not even let me hold her hand. She would not let me get to within 3 to 4 feet of her. No one had prepped us for anything like this. This is common with morphine.

<u>That was the absolute worst period of my entire life.</u> Morphine and drugs can do horrible things. I didn't know what to do. Around 4 AM the nurse told me to go home and get some rest. Both of you should admit early on your spouse will realize at some point what is happening.

Doctor's note @ 9:27 AM on Wednesday 6/5

Patient more agitated and delirious overnight. Today recognizes me and says **"Stop all this. Let me go."** Had emotional interaction with husband last night. Patient was delirious accusing everybody in the unit of trying to kill her, including her husband. She kept pulling the O2 mask off, will treat her delirium with haldon to insure her safety. (No one ever told me about this. The medical community will love you to death. I have some 160 pages of these. I found out about this information six weeks after Nancy's death. You can have access by just asking. Ask the doctors. JMC).

**You need "let me go. It's OK" statements. It is taken care of. Prayer. If you stay, it's great. If you go, we will miss you, but God wants you. The following came from others. Will you wait on me? I will wait on you. Mom and I will wait on you. I will miss you forever ... until I see you again. Start now on a page of "final words". Then review them early on with each other.

It was too late for Nancy and me to have had any conversation by this time. Again, we never got a chance to say good bye, no final hug, nothing after almost 53 years of marriage. She still had days to go.

You should know what your spouse will want for comfort and support. You should discuss this in great detail. Take a close look at these notes. They may give you some ideas. I suggest talking to your pastor and/or hospice people months early. If you don't talk this out the survivor is going to feel really, really bad and/or guilty for years to come! No one needs to carry this guilt around. If you feel any guilt, no matter what, you will need to learn how to forgive yourself. I can only warn the readers. I'm still working through my mine. I hope time will blunt the pain.

10:00 AM Wed. YES 3 TIMES. When her brother, a pastor, arrived, he quickly heard her anger. She said "I'm so angry with him!" She was full of non-specific accusation. Her brother tried to understand what it was that was troubling her so very much, but her mind couldn't focus enough to let her say anything that he could grasp. Giving up on trying to discern what it was that she was so upset about, he told her that just as we were forgiven by God unconditionally because of the blood Jesus shed for our sins, Jesus had called all of His followers to also forgive one another in the same way. She softened some. She stated "yes" strongly three times when her brother asked her three times if she believed in

Christ, but still declared her anger. I heard her. Nancy's anger had begun to reduce.

I then left her room so that her brother could speak with her privately. He later told me that he again went over the simple truth of the forgiveness for all people who turn to Jesus. After a few more seconds of consideration, she said, "That's right, I have to forgive him." Sounds just like Nancy. Faithful, logical and blunt to the end. Faith is a wonderful thing. Her brother told me that he prayed with her for the desire to forgive, reminding her that I loved her very much and that if God had forgiven me for every sin in my life, she surely could also forgive me. Colossians 3:13-14 forgiveness, 3:19 bitterness.

I then returned to the room, and her countenance had relaxed and with peace in her voice and on her face, she turned to me and told me "I forgive you" and she let me hold her hand again as she waited for God to take her. <u>Her forgiving me was the absolute best moment of my life</u>. Later that day she told me "I love you". What a wonderful blessing from a giving woman. Those were the last words she was ever able to say to me. <u>This was the greatest gift of my life</u>. You will find comfort in the future if you have something of this nature to remember. Over the next days there were times her eyes would follow me, but she was unable to make a sentence. I wish that I had known then what you are learning now. I imagine it took quite an effort for her to get those last three words out. What was going on in her mind? Again, we never got a chance to say good bye, no final hug, nothing after almost 53 years of marriage. She still had days to go.

To me, this book is a reading requirement for all Christians. "HEAVEN - Your Real Home". Joni Eareckson Tada. Both of you please read this way before your loved one goes into final weeks/days. It is only about 200 pages. If you do this it will help both of you. I would summarize Nancy during this period as confused, frustrated, afraid and angry. Her conscious world over the last two months had shrunk to a day or two then down to hours. When you get very ill this can happen. The spouse will need to adjust. You will too. The book will help.

Also, after much more reading and soul searching I found another thing we should have done. I had provided as much physical comfort for Nancy as I knew how to. I have realized now that by concentrating on just physically supporting her we put off confronting the total reality of death. I believe this could been another reason for her confusion in intensive care. She didn't know and didn't like it. Possibly, if we had discussed the actual process of her death, combined with her faith and had developed a complete understanding of how and when she could "let go" on her own terms, her passing could have been a blessing. Make heavy use of the church, hospice, family and the medical community way, way, way before you get this far. Bring them all deeply into the final journey on this earth.

June 6, 2013 Thurs. By this time the bacteria cultures had come back. The Docs told me all they could do would be to start the cultures all over again. They did not know what else to do. This would take a minimum of five days with little hope of success or survival. Nancy and I had known her doctor for more than 15 years. He had tears in his eyes when he told me this. Good man. He played third base and I played second base. We split short stop. I think we should have put her in hospice at that point. All the observable infection was clearing by now. Knee and port. Did the Docs realize at that time, the sepsis bacteria had destroyed the capability of her lungs and cardiovascular system to recover? I was never told. By now 97+% of the time she was unconscious.

Nancy was a Christian woman of great faith. She knew God was waiting for her. I believe she was tired of fighting and wanted to go home to Him. <u>During this period I made the most difficult decision I have ever made.</u> I quit asking God to keep her on this earth, and began to pray for God to take her home to heaven. I know it was the correct decision, but I felt like it almost killed me.

FRIDAY 6/7/2013 START

I will cover Friday and Saturday with various Doctor's Notes only. Nancy's status continued to deteriorate. I am using this format to give the reader a more detailed picture of the information you can access.

Filed: 6/7/2013 7:58

General appearance - acutely ill, fatigued. Subjective: Rested more comfortably last night.

1. Worsening respiratory failure - suspect multifactorial possible pneumonia - empiric treatment for PCP, GNRs, GPCs
2. Port infection s/p line removal - site improving (very much so. Too late now. Sepsis has done its damage to Nancy's lungs. JMC)
3. Left knee cellulitis improved

Physical Exam: Color good. Lethargic but interactive; Lungs sound clearer, better airflow. Skin Lesions about the same.

Single view chest. Indication: Pneumonia. IMPRESSION: Persistent bilateral airspace disease slightly worse over the right lower lobe. Findings: Compared to examination dated 6/6/2013, the right upper extremity PICC remains in place. Mild reticulonodular opacity over both upper lungs remains. Aeration may be slightly better, however, over the right lung base, airspace opacity is denser suggesting interval worsening. There is persistent dense opacity over the left base as well. There may be very small pleural effusions. Cardiomediastinal contours are stable. Overall lung aeration is stable to slightly worse. No neumothorax. The bony thorax is otherwise unremarkable.

Filed: 6/7/2013 8:03 AM Note Time: 6/7/2013 7:56 AM

Hematologic/Infectious- Continue broad spectrum antimicrobial coverage, cultures negative to date.

Decision Making -DNR / MPOA on chart / We will not escalate to level of care at this time (e.g. no BIPAP). If there is no significant improvement by 6/8 AM, likely will transfer to hospice care center. The patients 3 children with be arriving from out of town 6/8 PM. Appreciate Dr. xx's support.

Dr. xx. No pathology/cultures to clarify what is making the difference, but signs of improvement; Still a long way to go. I sensed the family was leaning toward Palliative Care or home by tomorrow depending on the level of care/treatment we continue; ...but I would consider: See how today goes, and how family feels, - with signs of improvement in the last two days, that we give her the best supportive chance to recover, And continue current input treatment through the weekend, and see if progress continues -- still emphasizing comfort and not uncomfortable procedures, and clarify duration, and which Abx, etc. Spent 35 minutes time in patient care.

Over 50% of this time was in counseling and coordination of care.

Meanwhile continue Antibiotics, and increase comfort measures, at risk of declining pulmonary condition. Spent 60 minutes time in patient care. Over 50% of this time was in counseling and coordination of care. Using the same lesion on her right leg, as this looked safest lesion to obtain with patient cooperation level. Sent for G Stain, cultres for bacteria, AFB and fungal. In saline guaze soaked container to not dry out. Response to therapy thus far has been poor - while cellulitic lesion improve new ecchymotic ones develop

Physical Exam:

Filed: 6/7/2013 10:42

24 Hour Events:

Confusion improved. (Hard to show confusion when you can't talk JMC)

Worse respiratory status. Neurologic-Confusion and delirium improved. Trial of oral pain med for longer duration of relief metabolic encephalopathy. Negative MRI brain

Cardiac/Hemodynamic-Severe sepsis.

Respiratory -oxygen requirements slightly increased. Chest x-ray with worse consolidation in base

Discussed with husband at bedside and outside of room to discuss end of life management if patient does not improve.

Last data filed at 06/07/13 2200 Physical Exam: General appearance - acutely ill, dyspnea Chest - decreased air entry noted throughout, coarse crackles, and rapid respiratory rate. (I think God let Nancy stay with us in order to say goodbye to the kids the next day when they came in from out of town. JMC)

Patient Goals: comfort, would want to go home if able. (hospice eligible) (No one told me this.)

Palliative Care Daily Progress Note

Current Code Status: DNR. (I asked about increasing oxygen input. The damage to her lungs and cardiovascular system was so bad by this time the 02 would not be able to go into the blood stream. JMC) 6/7/2013 END FRIDAY

(3) Hospice location

Note; you may have problems concentrating by this point. Preplanning will be a great help.

Where are the "hospice" activities to take place? Nancy would have rather been at home. No one told me this. I found out six weeks later while reviewing the Doctors Notes.

When does someone tell you of the options? I don't remember being given any options. I believe all anyone wanted me to do was sign contracts for payments.

Where are you going to put the medical bed in your home? Plan ahead.

Where does the medical support come from? What happens if they are not there when you need them?

When and how is it set up?

Contact names and telephone/cell #s.

How is it paid for?

(4) Hospice care - No more Doctor's Notes from this point forward.

June 8, 2013 Sat. I had Nancy taken to palliative/hospice care about 8:30 PM. Her hospital ICU shift nurses came in and gave her hugs after her eight days in ICU as she was taken away. I did not see anyone else get this treatment. They all thought she was a sweetie. I remember following the ambulance. The sun had set.

As palliative care was setting her up (9:30 PM June 8)) all 3 kids quietly walked in. Somehow she awoke and said to Scott "what are you doing here?" How did she know they were there? That was the last firm, full sentence I heard Nancy say. Nancy had been comatose the prior 30 hours. By the grace of God her mind partially came back for about 20 to 30 minutes and her children got to talk a tad to their Mom.

Sherry said Nancy did ask her "did you find something for Tyler?" It was very difficult for Nancy to talk. Her lungs were shot by this time. Nancy was asking about Tyler's efforts to find an apartment in Boston where he was going to college. Sherry answered and told Nancy that Tyler was OK. Sherry went blank from that point forward. She did not remember anything more. Be prepared for this. Nancy did say she was thirsty. One of the kids brought her an iced lemon-line drink. Sandy also went blank and did not remember if Nancy even knew if she was there. Sandy did tell Nancy to breathe calmly. It would help like in child birth. She would forget about it. The nurses all agreed. Nancy came around enough to say "they lie". She could hear conversations. Her mind was still totally there. Hearing is one of the last things to go.

Her brother, Scott, said Sherry, oldest daughter, told Nancy she and Scott were going to leave and go to our home for sleep. Nancy told Sherry "good night". Nancy also told Scott "good night baby boy". Those may have been the last focused, cognizant words ever she said

We never got to talk to her again. We all took turns holding her hands 24/7. Did this have to take three days? Could we have started the process earlier? All the kids mentioned the glazed eyes and confusion. Nancy raised three wonderful kids. They got their Dad through the next week.

June 9, 2013 Sun By this time the antibiotics had totally killed the visible infections and her skin was healing. Her knee, the port surgery, the transfusion tube access point and other skin infection areas were almost clear. By early Monday morning her skin was smooth as a young woman, completely healed. This had to be one of the most incredible, wonderful things I have ever seen. It was too late for her body to repair the damage from the hurricane to her lungs and cardio vascular systems.

June 10, 2013 Mon The final Dr. (hospice) explained to me what had happened to Nancy. This was the last full day under full medical care. Why was I not told days earlier? Maybe Nancy could have been spared days of confusion, frustration and pain. I don't know. The Dr. said bacterial sepsis is like a hurricane. It can kill you in a matter of hours. Especially if you have a weak/compromised immune system.

Picture hurricane wind bands coming ashore. The wind surges knock everything down. Then the hurricane moves inshore and dies. When you go back to the path there is nothing left except total devastation. Nancy's devastation were her lungs and cardiovascular systems. All we could do was to let her pass as quietly as possible. The hospice people did good.

June 11, 2013 Tue.

Sandy was on one side of the bed and Scott on the other. I was across the room. I looked up and saw tears in Sandy's eyes. Scott stood up and said "Dad. It's happening. Come here". I took Nancy's left hand as she had wanted me to. I put my other hand on Nancy's left shoulder. Thank you son. Scott went and got Sherry and within two minutes we surrounded her. She took a few more very, very light, small, calm breaths. Her pulse, in her neck, gently faded and stopped. June 11, 2013 @ 5:15 PM. I lost Nancy to God as he took her to heaven exactly as Nancy had wished. Within 2 seconds, I swear, she looked 15 years younger. Totally relaxed. No more pain or confusion. No more strife. Only peace and comfort. I think Nancy would have liked the following quote. I would like it also at my time. I am not as strong in my faith as Nancy was. I work on it daily.

The time of my departure is at hand. I have fought the good fight. I have finished the race. I have kept the faith. Finally there is laid up for me the crown of righteousness, which the Lord, the righteous Judge, will give to me that day, and not to me only but also to all who will love His appearing. I hope I qualify for this. I know Nancy did.

(5) Lymphodema

This problem usually does not generate a lot of attention until it is too late. As you can tell from the preceding you will have to stay on top of it. The lymph system removes waste materials from the interstitial spaces (spaces between the cells) after the circulatory system delivers oxygen and nutrients. After the cells use the good stuff they kick the waste materials out into the interstitial spaces. The system functions like the slow moving river that runs through South Florida draining the Everglades swamp and the thousands of acres of cattle grazing lands and their excreta. When the system gets plugged up or overloaded it turns into a stagnant swamp. Bacteria will breed unless the swamp is cleared. Wet lands and people die.

The system is constructed like a series of pipes with one way valves. When you have muscular activity, the pressure pushes the liquid forward through the valves. More activity, more forward movement. Tiny pipes drain into small pipes which drain into larger pipes. There were times when Nancy's lower legs would pump up to where they felt almost a hard as a green pepper. Sooner or later, in a healthy person, the waste materials drain out. Simple when it works. When it did not, Nancy developed a deadly biological sepsis infection. I believe it started with a scratch in her garden about a week prior to her admittance to the emergency ward. Sepsis was listed on her death certificate. I had no idea. No one told me about all this. Now you know. Go back to May 15, 2013. Some of the primary causes/sources are soil, perhaps in a garden (you know what ends up in a garden) and hospitals.

There are both manual and mechanical compression methods to assist the lymph system. You can learn to do it yourself. You can find all sorts of information by accessing the web. As already mentioned a person with a compromised immune system can develop sepsis and pass away in hours. The following is a guess. I think Nancy had at least 35 to 40 pounds of liquid drained in the eleven days she was in the hospitals. Can you imagine what her lymph system looked like? There were times weeks before that she could have a tiny scratch on a leg and the clear liquid would literally actually ooze from a nonvisible scratch.

(6) Morphine

This section is difficult to reconcile with what I saw to what information I have been able to locate. If you can find supportable information we could add it to this section. Remember everyone reacts differently.

A good source so far has been: Hospicefoundation.org. Myths about pain (end of life) was a real good section. It goes along with what happened to Nancy. When going on-line it appears that every source is trying to at least subtly trying sell you something. Many of the sites suggest help from an anesthesiologist or a pain relief specialist. This is a VERY good move. During some circumstances morphine can depress the respiratory system. It appears to still be considered the most effective drug for pain although there are many people that react very poorly to it. Morphine dulls the senses. It is a pain blocker. It rarely promotes total relief.

There are more types of substitutes than I can count. Here are some: hydromorphone, tramadol, oxycodone (many brand names) oxymorphan, fentanyl, levorphanol, methadone, panadol, voltaren, demerol, toradol, diaudid. Don't be afraid to stand up for yourself

Armageddon

One of the series "Left Behind" books, number 11, pages 161 through 162" presents what I and others have gone through with the impacts of morphine. As I was reading I was stunned at how close it was to what happened to me and Nancy and others I have talked to. One of the authors must have had the same experience. I too spoke harshly in anger and confusion to Nancy June 5th at 2:30 AM when she was having problems with the oxygen mask. The only time in 52 plus years. That may have pushed her into her anger with me. I may never know. I handled the delirium problem poorly. You need to talk to someone that has been there.

(7) Early life style changes

This is probably too late for your sufferer now, but.... maybe you can head off cancer/heart problems for someone else. These items change relative positions every year. They still show up every year. They all have the probability of causing disease. 1) Smoking, 2) too heavy (fat) 3) lack of exercise and 4) too much alcohol consumption.

I truly think that by making early changes in her life style Nancy could have survived. Here is why. One of the first tests that was given after the diagnosis of multiple myeloma was to check the condition and capacity of her lungs. Nancy had been a smoker starting at age 15 and smoked sporadically her whole life. She quit immediately after the cancer diagnosis. She walked out onto the back porch, threw the cigarette into the butt can, and said "no more." She never looked back. She still missed smoking. The lung test showed a loss of 30 to 40 percent of lung capacity never to be recovered. With the full complement of alveoli in her lungs, could she have survived? The capacity and damage test is quite inexpensive.

(8) Oximeter

This is another item Nancy has given. Some people reading this will experience what we did. We could have known earlier that she was fading. Get the Dr. to explain to you the function and use of a pulse oximeter. Should not take 15 minutes. Cost about $34.00 at Walmart.

What impact will O2 deprivation have? Sometimes enough oxygen can-not go into the blood stream. What is the problem? Get an understandable explanation.

Limp extremities. Define C02 poisoning. What does it feel like to the patient? Limpness starts in the extremities and works inward - just like hypothermia - go to sleep. What do you look for?

Color of finger nails and skin.

Correct use of the Pulse/02 unit.

Remember tachypnea: Rapid breathing > 20 breaths per minute. Nancy got up to about 70 per minute.

When do they start breathing more gently?

How much time is left?

Who stays when you have to sleep? You will want to be there when your spouse passes. Who is responsible to wake you up? A friend of mine whose wife was in hospice went home to fix dinner and about twenty minutes later they called to tell of his wife's death. Made him really angry. Nothing he could do. He wanted to be with her.

Had we known what the oximeter was telling us the last 15 to 20 minutes we would have talked her to heaven. I do not know if she was conscious enough to hear and understand us. Remember, hearing is one of the last senses to go. The girls had just finished washing her hands and arms and brushing her hair. They had put lotion on her skin for dryness abatement. I checked her with the oximeter. It was "winking", not pulsing steadily. One of the daughters said that perhaps the lotion was interfering. Then it quit working. Nancy was still breathing and appeared to be relaxed and perhaps asleep. We didn't know that Nancy was preparing to depart this world. If we had known we could have told her that we were all there by name. That we were physically holding her hands and shoulders in case God was getting ready to take her to heaven just as Nancy had wanted me to do. We could have told her individually, by name, one last time that we loved her.

Bereavement

The following are from various sources. They are the best items I have found. "Most people who suffer a loss experience one or more of the following items, which are all natural and normal grief responses.

* Feelings of tightness in the throat or heaviness in the chest.
* An empty feeling in the stomach and loss of appetite.
* Feel guilty at times and angry with others.
* Feel restless and look for activity, but find it difficult to concentrate.

* Feel as though the loss is not real; that it really didn't happen.
* Sense the loved one's presence, seeing, hearing, starting to talk to them.
* Wander aimlessly. What am I doing? Forget and don't finish what you have started.
* Have difficulty sleeping and dream of their loved one frequently.
* Assume mannerisms or traits of their loved one.
* Experience an intense preoccupation with the life of the deceased. Memories.
* Feel guilty or angry over things that happened or did not happen in the relationship.
* Feel intensely angry with the loved one for leaving them.
* Feel as though you need to take care of people who seem uncomfortable around you by not talking about the feelings of loss.
* Need to tell and retell and remember things about the loved one and the experience of their death.
* Feel mood changes over the slightest things. Startling and surprising.
* Cry at unexpected times. Crashing grief.

Remember: being correct or knowing what you are doing will not make the lonelies disappear or explain why God left you here when half your life is already in heaven. My opinion: try not to live in the past.

Summary

Nancy gave her life to me and she was always there for me to come home to for 52 years and 9 months. As I write this, December 2013, we all celebrate Christmas and the fact that Nancy is in a different, better home. I look forward to seeing her there. As a matter of fact, we are all welcome there. We can have coffee together.

Hopefully this information will help focus your attention in order to get you into the mental shape you may need during this time. If there is information, changes, deletions, additions that would help anyone else, locate me and please e-mail. We can use it for the next release.

110+ TO-DO ITEMS

(1) Prior to death: To-Do's

There are times you may feel helpless. These items will at least give you something to do that will keep you busy. There a number of these that will take a doctor's input. Initial and date every activity as you complete it. I found a good word after Nancy's death. The word is "beloved". Wish I had found it much earlier.

Psalms 90:12.Teach us to number our days carefully that we may develop wisdom in our hearts. Remember; share a last kiss and hug while you know they are still cognizant.

If your spouse likes to dance - learn how. Right now!

OK _____

Keep a large work/appointment calendar. Tie to diary. 16"x20".

OK _____

Keep a diary, medical dates and knowledge items

OK _____

Set up your 3 ring binder for CBC, doctor, hospital and hospice reports

OK _____

Set up a contacts book

Medicare, Medicaid, VA, Soc. Sec., private insurers, qualified support, friends support, Church, doctors, clinics, insurer names, account ID's, policy numbers, contacts. Investments, attorneys, executor, etc. tel. numbers, email, etc.

OK _____

Let the patient know you are thinking about them when you can't be there. Family, friends, etc. Letters, text, and make calls.

OK _____

Will: copies and distribution. Does the executor consent to do this function? Do they know what is required?

OK _____

Distribution of personal items

OK _____ See last page.

Where is the jewelry? Who gets it?

OK _____

There will probably be times for physical therapy. Go with them. Could be exercise, walking, etc.

OK _____

When you get the bad news notify everyone concerned immediately. Family, friends, doctors, etc.

OK _____

Assist with cooking, cleaning baths, making beds, moping, mowing yard, driving, etc.

OK _____

Food: simple to complex. Need recipes. The fellows will probably struggle here. The cooking spouse should start teaching the other spouse a LOT about cooking. Nancy did this for me. She was very subtle. I did not know she was teaching me. The non-cooking spouse should take over this duty, 100 percent, for at least one day a week.

OK _____

Get some good pictures: individual, together and family. Your memories will fade.

OK _____

Last care wishes

      Copies to doctors   OK_____
      Copies to hospital   OK _____
      Care givers   OK _____
      At home location   OK _____

Grave plot purchase

OK _____

Cremation, vault, coffin, ashes final container, where to dispose, sprinkle, etc.

OK _____

Do not resuscitate band. Check with hospital where to get one.

OK _____

Grave stone/monument: material, color, texture, wording, height, width, thickness, shape, font, font sizes, cost, delivery and set up details, scheduling and contacts. Nancy and I put "Traveling Buddies" at the bottom of our stone. A cross was placed in the middle.

OK _____

Driver's license: organ donor, medical/drug requirements. Blood type, veteran's status, special driving requirements. All states are different.

OK _____

Weight vs. chemicals. Lymph system. What to do about it. See Section #2.

OK _____

Talk about hair loss with chemo. Everyone will get used to it.

OK _____

Have doctor define bacterial and viral infection. Have them explain what to look for. Inflammation, localized heat, swelling, weakness, signs of oxygen deprivation (see oximeter Section #2) unable or unwilling to stay awake, problems finishing sentences.

OK _____

Will the rings be easy to remove? I had to have Nancy's resized the year before she passed.

OK _____

Prayers: for healing (go to your earthly home?) or for death (go to your home in heaven?)

What does your spouse want? Are they able to participate?

OK _____

How strong is their faith? Should you ask them? When?

OK _____

Nancy and I never asked each other how strong the other's faith was. The joy of the Lord was her strength. Mine too. You will get through it. You have no choice.

Should you pray together? Should you hold hands?

OK _____

What do you do if your spouse develops shakes at home? What temperature ranges are acceptable? When do you take them to the emergency ward?

OK _____

_____

_____

_____

Actions required if the spouse passes out at home?

OK _____

_____

_____

_____

Report any rash or infection to your emergency support team immediately.

OK _____

_____

_____

_____

Report any temperature spikes to you emergency support team immediately.

OK _____

_____

_____

_____

Notification lists in/out of town.

OK _____

Take food to others while you can. They will appreciate it and remember the patient to the survivor. Nancy loved to do this for others.

OK _____

Tuck the loved on into bed. Then you can go out and watch TV.

OK _____

Call and have final word with old friends.

Name: _____ OK _____
Name: _____ OK _____
Name: _____ OK _____
Name: _____ OK _____

Who is going to teach you to understand the start and ongoing impact of (heart) pulmonary, (lung) alveoli problems? How bad is it? Is it lack of O2 in each blood cell or lack of blood cells or both? Is it the problem of O2 getting into the blood stream? What are the doctors doing to fix the problem? What is the prognosis?

OK _____

Are you going to keep your spouse alive if there is no chance of success? (See legal info.) Should Anyone have the option to choose the time, place, surroundings and method of their death?

OK _____

Look for open, comprehending eyes. Use for communication opportunities. Use hand squeezes as a method of communicating.

OK _____

How does the entry of extraordinary measures fit here?

OK _____

Impact of morphine. Delirium. What do you do when the spouse goes into delirium? How do you react, talk to them, hold them and support them?

OK _____

Impact of MEDS. What meds? What are they? What do they do? Keep in front of your medical log.

OK _____

Hearing is one of the last senses to go. We could tell she was with us till the last few hours. How do you know? Does everyone understand this? No arguments in front of the patient.

OK _____

So much can happen in a short period of time you both may become very tired: physically, mentally, emotionally and spiritually. Share with your support group.

OK _____

What are their favorite songs? Nancy's was Amazing Grace. I did not know this until she was in intensive care. List top three here.

_____

_____

_____

OK _____

Digestive system shuts down. When? How do you know? What does this mean? Can you or should you give water, food or 02? This will be a concern to you.

OK _____

_____

_____

_____

Get doctors to give odds and time frames. Some dislike doing this. Pressure them. I failed to do this. That was an omission on my part. You have to know what is going on if you are going to take care of them.

OK _____

Do you know how often the patient need to be turned? Every RN seems to have a different idea.

OK _____

Talk about your loved one's last human touch and what they want to hear from you. See memorial comments. No medical person mentioned a final hug, or kiss, or I love you. I missed eleven days of final affection - both in ICU and hospice.

OK _____

Do they want you to hold their hand, rub their back or shoulders? Most do. Check for dry lips and throat .They will probably want water or ice cubes.

OK _____

Get medical support to explain what the "death rattle" means and sounds like. This is another tough one. Really tough. I would not review this with anyone less than sixteen years old unless they are going to be there at the end. It does not always happen.

OK _____

(2) After death to-do's

The survivor is going to literally dismantle the spouse's life. The process will probably be very emotionally difficult.

The survivor will need to know about the following activities. Get the Spouse to show you about these items while still able to do so. Identify where all the records are located; accounts, statements, warrantees, etc.

Use washing machine, dish washer, clean porcelain sink vs. stainless steel, ironing, etc.

      OK _____

How often do I clean the bath room(s)? What with? Learn about bleach.

      OK _____

Exterior window and screen cleaning, materials locations

      OK _____

Lawn mower and sprinkler operation and maintenance.

      Ok _____

Check book(s). Where are records located? Learn how to manage accounts. Write checks and/or use electronic payments, balance and reconcile. Tie to credit cards.

      OK _____

Check book(s) change/review all access names. Set how long in future to close out and remove signers. Get advice from your banker. See your contacts book.

      OK _____

Investments. Get contact names, telephone and e-mail numbers. See your contacts book.

OK _____

Wills, trusts, beneficiaries, copies, locations, executor assigned and ready to go to work.

OK _____

Location(s) _____

_____

Executor _____

_____

Auto titles. May need to change these. What is required to sell one in your state?

OK _____

Social Security. Call and set up the appointment to close out records. Most are nice people.

OK _____

Telephone use, security codes, remote and out of state bank access. I was lost on these items.

OK _____ See your contacts book.

Obituary w/picture(s). Run for more than one day. See samples Section #2. Who is going to write it? Nancy and I both started early. We used newspaper examples to help us. I got mine done. Nancy got about 15 % done. She could not face it. The kids took over and finished it after she died.

OK _____

Church announcements. I forgot to follow up. There were some that missed Nancy's memorial. They let me know about it in no uncertain terms. They were embarrassed when they saw me and did not know what had happened.

OK _____

Memorial thank you notes. I never thought of this.

OK _____

Final memorial process. Who does what? Do you want a canned pitch? I have seen a few where the presenter obviously had no idea about who he was talking about. Songs? Bible readings. I had no clue what Nancy wanted. You may not want any of this. I did the following steps at Nancy's memorial. Some people just can't handle this job.

1) Pastor's introduction and Bible verse reading. What is their favorite bible passage? Then he read a wonderful letter written by Nancy's best friend.
2) We sang "Amazing Grace", her favorite song. Then I read "I Will Rise". Someone may like to use these songs. Nancy's second favorite song was "Wings Of A Dove". No one knew this one except Nancy. Ferlin Husky - 1960. These are included in Section #1.Then I read the BUCKET LIST from Section #1. The congregation had asked for these items. It was pretty rough. Very few dry eyes. This took about a half hour.
3) Then Nancy's brother, a pastor, told some funny stories about his little sister. Thank you brother. That was really wonderful. He lightened the atmosphere.
4) The pastor closed out. We all sat for lunch. There were so many people we had to go get more chairs. A number of people came to me later and said "we needed that". This is when the Nancy Notes started.

OK _____

Flowers. Start early. Take pictures. The florist forgot to do this. Our kids never got to see their mom's flowers. What colors, type, presentation?

OK _____

Death certificate. How many 10+. I have used as many as 20 as executor.

OK _____

Bring family in. Flights, auto rental, motels, etc. Get help from family members. You will probably be pretty frazzled by this point.

OK _____

Who cleans out the deceased's stuff? Do not do this by yourself. Use family, friends, church etc. You will find items that will tug at your heart. Take your time. Consider charities.

OK _____

Sell the house. Selling a home is beyond Nancy Notes.

OK _____

Auto, fire, life, disability and health policies. Close and change names.

OK _____

Close our doctors, dentists, ophthalmologists, etc. if you are moving or changing.

OK _____

Is the survivor going to leave town? Where are you going? Why? You can dicker with movers.

OK _____

Does the survivor have a living plan? (I got this from a pastor) Have you considered a companion or marriage? How are you going to find someone? Have you discussed this with your spouse? I never thought of it. Did Nancy? You have no idea how lonely it can be. I understand it can be rougher on the fellows than the girls.

    OK _____

MEMORANDUM FOR DISPOSITION OF TANGIBLE PERSONAL PROPERTY

Pursuant to the terms of my Will dated August 10, 2007, I have requested the distribution of certain items of my tangible personal property in accordance with a writing or memorandum, and this memorandum is made for such purpose. If the named beneficiary of a particular item does not survive me by more than thirty days, such item shall be disposed of as though it has not been listed herein.

Description of Item	Name of Beneficiary
Oak icebox	Sandra L. Keeton
Oak school desk w/wrought iron legs	Sandra L. Keeton
Nanny's small 3 slat hard oak rocker	James Scott Coston
Granner's magazine rack painted occasional table	James Scott Coston
4 quite small western oils by Aunt Doris Greenacre	Sherry C. Novak
Cousin Blanch Albright's primitive oil of Daniel's Park area	James Scott Coston
Jim's charcoal drawing of trees	James Scott Coston
Jim's watercolor tree – green	Sandra L. Keeton
Jim's 2 Navy service plaques	James Scott Coston
Step-stool made by Great-grandfather Reed	Sherry C. Novak
Oak glass front china cabinet	Sandra L. Keeton
Oak dining table, 6 straight back chairs	James Scott Coston
Nanny's glass globe lamp	Sherry C. Novak
Nanny's Singer sewing machine	Sherry C. Novak
Noritaki china	James Scott Coston
Nanny's round (oak?) lamp table	Sandra L. Keeton
Granner's maple secretary	Sherry C. Novak
Old framed greeting cards	Sherry C. Novak
Oak Hall tree	Sherry C. Novak
2 ink reprints by High Museum of Art maintenance supervisor	James Scott Coston
Cedar chest made by Great-grandfather Reed	Sherry C. Novak
3 drawer oak dresser w/rectangular Tilt attached mirror	Sandra L. Keeton
3 drawer & 1 door oak washstand table	Sandra L. Keeton
Oak Victorian replication carved queen bed frame	James Scott Coston
5 drawer oak chest –of-drawers	James Scott Coston
3 drawer oak dresser w/square tilt attached mirror	James Scott Coston
27½ "x 17½" oak mirror	James Scott Coston
Gilt framed round mirror	Sherry C. Novak
2 oval pictures (one is of Bess Reed Coston)	Sherry C. Novak
Oak marble top dresser w/43"x34" separate mirror (Nanny's)	Sherry C. Novak
Oak marble top washstand table (Nanny's)	Sherry C. Novak
Cedar 2 door (one w/mirror) oddity (Great-grandfather Reed)	Sherry C. Novak
Oak queen spindle bed	Sandra L. Keeton
Leffert's dark (Oak?) bench	Sandra L. Keeton
5 serving pieces Haviland China (Dram's)	James Scott Coston
China teacup collection (17) & cream & sugars (3)	Sherry C. Novak

Signature _____

Printed in the United States
By Bookmasters